New Year Detox

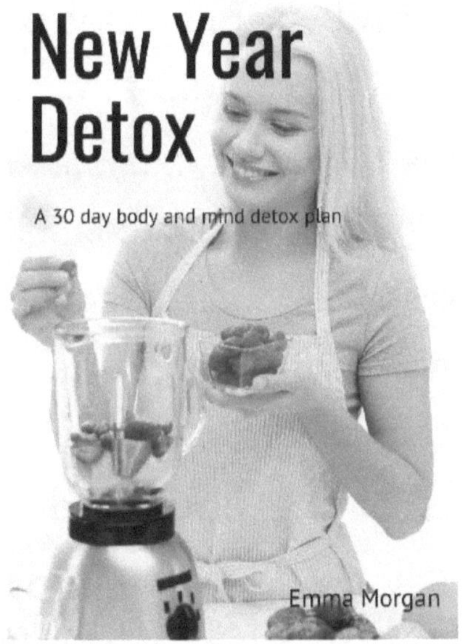

A 30-Day Body and Mind Detox Blueprint

New Year Detox

A 30-Day Body and Mind Detox Blueprint

Contents

New Year Detox

A 30-Day Body and Mind Detox Blueprint

New Year Detox

A 30-Day Body and Mind Detox Blueprint

New Year Detox

A 30-Day Body and Mind Detox Blueprint

New Year Detox

A 30-Day Body and Mind Detox Blueprint

Copyright and Enquiries

Comments or enquiries may be left in the Aging Slowdown *Contact Us* page at

https://agingslowdown.com/contact-us/

New Year Detox

A 30-Day Body and Mind Detox Blueprint

Disclaimer

Please note the information contained within this document is for educational and entertainment purposes only. Every attempt has been made to provide accurate, up to date, reliable and complete information. No warranties of any kind are expressed or implied. Readers acknowledge that the author is not engaging in the rendering of legal, financial, medical or professional advice.

By reading this document, the reader agrees that under no circumstances are we responsible for any losses, direct or indirect, which are incurred as a result of the use of information contained within this document, including, but not limited to, errors, omissions, or inaccuracies.

New Year Detox

Introduction

Detoxes have become increasingly popular in recent years. By removing toxins from your body via detox, you can boost your overall health, increase your energy levels, reduce your risk of chronic disease and much more.

However, many modern detox programs focus exclusively on detoxing the body and neglect the mind. As a result, negative thoughts and stress can still have a detrimental impact on your mental and physical wellbeing while completing these detoxes.

The Body and Mind Detox Blueprint addresses this problem by providing you with a selection of weekly practices that you can use to eliminate toxic thoughts from your mind and remove toxic substances from your body. In this eBook we'll provide you with:

- An overview of the **Body and Mind Detox Blueprint**
- A list of the benefits you can enjoy by completing the **Body and Mind Detox Blueprint**
- A detailed **Body and Mind Detox Blueprint** that provides you with specific actions to cleanse your body and mind

Although the Body and Mind Detox Blueprint can benefit you at any time, it's a great way to start off a new year. That's why this book is called New Year Detox.

New Year Detox

The Body and Mind Detox Blueprint Overview

As mentioned above, **The Body and Mind Detox Blueprint** provides you with a detailed action plan that contains specific actions you can use to eliminate mental and physical toxins from your life. These actions are broken down into four weekly segments and then the program finishes with a two day liquid and mind detox.

The last two days of **The Body and Mind Detox Blueprint** involve drinking just juice and spending lots of time alone to fully cleanse your body and mind. Therefore, it's advisable to plan your 30-day detox so that the last two days fall on a weekend or on days where you have no other commitments.

The section below provides further details on each part of **The Body and Mind Detox Blueprint**:

Week 1 (Days 1-7)

The first week of The Body and Mind Detox Blueprint involves:

Body Detox: Eliminating alcohol and processed foods from your diet.

Mind Detox: Avoiding the news, reducing your exposure to light at night and learning to say no.

New Year Detox

This first week removes hundreds of harmful toxins from your lifestyle. It also removes a lot of negativity and stress from your mind and enhances your sleep quality.

Week 2 (Days 8-14)

The second week of The Body and Mind Detox Blueprint involves:

Body Detox: Eliminating caffeine and dairy from your diet.

Mind Detox: Avoiding social media, removing night time noise and spending time alone in nature.

This second week eliminates toxins that affect your digestion, energy levels and sleep quality. It will also calm your mind and help you feel more peaceful.

Week 3 (Days 15-21)

The third week of The Body and Mind Detox Blueprint involves:

Body Detox: Adding smoothies to your diet while also eliminating grains and starch.

Mind Detox: Limiting your Internet activity, going to bed at a fixed time and trying aromatherapy.

This third week boosts your digestive system by providing it with lots of essential nutrients while also eliminating carbohydrates that can have a negative impact on your blood glucose levels. It will enhance the sense of calm and peace that you developed in the previous week and further improve your sleep quality.

New Year Detox

Week 4 (Days 22-28)

The fourth week of The Body and Mind Detox Blueprint involves:

Body Detox: Adding juices to your diet while also eliminating meat.

Mind Detox: Stopping watching TV, developing a nightly bedtime ritual and trying meditation.

This fourth week further boosts your digestive system by adding nutrient rich juices and removing difficult to digest meats. It also removes a major source of mental distraction from your life (TV) and helps you achieve deep and full relaxation through meditation.

Days 29-30

The final two days of The Body and Mind Detox Blueprint involve:

Body Detox: Drinking just juice for the full two days.

Mind Detox: Completely disconnecting from technology and focusing fully on relaxation.

This is the most intensive part of the program but also the most rewarding. These final two days will leave you feeling fully cleansed, both mentally and physically.

New Year Detox

The Benefits of the Body and Mind Detox Blueprint

The Body and Mind Detox Blueprint has many mental and physical benefits and these are outlined below:

Benefit 1 – Improved Digestive Health

One of the biggest benefits of detoxing is that it allows clearing out your digestive system to give it time to rest and recharge. This improves the efficiency of your digestive system after the detox and allows you to extract more energy and nutrition from the foods you eat and to process waste materials more effectively.

Benefit 2 – Better Quality Sleep

Quality sleep is something that many of us don't get enough of. We often stay up late and don't get the required hours of sleep we need each night. In addition to this, we usually sleep in an environment that doesn't promote quality sleep.

The Body and Mind Detox Blueprint includes weekly practices that specifically focus on sleep quality. As a result, you'll be able to enjoy the deepest, most restful nights of sleep that you've ever experienced during this detox program.

Benefit 3 – Enhanced Energy Levels

Cutting foods out of your diet and replacing solid foods with juices and smoothies may sound like something that will leave you feeling tired, lethargic and lacking in energy.

However, detoxes often have the opposite effect and you're likely to find that you feel more alert, energetic and vibrant during your detox.

Benefit 4 – Greater Mental Clarity

Removing physical toxins from your body doesn't just improve your physical health. It also has a positive effect on your mind and enhances your awareness, concentration and focus. When combined with the mind detox elements of **The Body and Mind Detox Blueprint**, you'll find that you reach a level of mental clarity that you've never experienced before. This mental clarity will stay with you long after you finish the detox and greatly improve the quality of your thoughts.

Benefit 5 – Healthier Skin

The amount of toxins in your body has a direct influence on the health of your skin. When your body is full of toxins, your skin will look and feel dull, dry and lifeless. You'll also be more prone to skin disorders such as acne, eczema, or psoriasis. By completing a detox, you'll find that your skin completely transforms and becomes bright, smooth and clear.

Benefit 6 – Healthy, Long Term Weight Loss

One of the most underappreciated benefits of detox diets is that they promote healthy, long term weight loss. The dietary changes that you make during **The Body and Mind Detox Blueprint** will blast through body fat and help you lose weight. However, the habits that you develop over the

30 days will ensure that you don't put this weight back on. The increased mental clarity and awareness that you can get from the detox will make you more mindful of your eating choices and guide you towards healthy foods while the dietary changes that you make during the detox will likely lead to permanent improvements in the quality of foods that you eat.

Benefit 7 – Increased Happiness

Negativity is something that many of us fail to recognize in our daily lives. However, when we stop and listen to our internal dialogue, it's rarely positive and is often full of cruel, negative, destructive thoughts. The messages that we receive through the Internet, TV, social media and even those around us can greatly add to this negativity and detract from our happiness and wellbeing.

The Body and Mind Detox Blueprint directly removes these negative influences from your life and incorporates a range of techniques that help you relax and feel more positive including aromatherapy and meditation. The overall result is that during the 30 days your happiness levels will greatly improve and you'll be able to maintain this elevated level of happiness after you complete the detox.

Benefit 8 – Improved Immunity

The toxins that build up in your body have a negative effect on your immune system and inhibit its ability to fight disease, illness and infection. By eliminating these toxins through a detox, you'll be able to restore your immune system and maximize its effectiveness.

Benefit 9 – Protection Against Chronic Disease

Stress and toxins are two of the leading risk factors for multiple types of chronic disease including cancer, heart disease and high blood pressure. **The Body and Mind Detox Blueprint** eliminates both of these risk factors by removing physical toxins from your body and providing you with techniques that you can use to release stress from your lifestyle.

Benefit 10 – Reduced Stress Levels

Stress is something that has become increasingly prevalent in our modern lives. With work, friends, family and technology all constantly placing demands on our time, it's very easy to start feeling stressed and overwhelmed. Not only do these stressful thoughts have a negative impact on our mental wellbeing and the way we feel but they can also be physically damaging to our bodies.

With **The Body and Mind Detox Blueprint**, you'll learn to identify the negative factors in your life that cause stress and distance yourself from them. Not only will this provide you with the break you need to rest, relax and de-stress but it will also help you to permanently lower your stress levels after you've completed the 30 day detox.

The Body and Mind Detox Blueprint – Week 1

The first week of **The Body and Mind Detox Blueprint** involves a total of five habit changes. The recommended approach is to change one habit for each of the first five days and then spend the final two days of the week practicing all five habits and making sure they stick. However, you can be flexible with your approach and use any techniques that best allow you to master these five habit changes by the end of the first week.

Habit Change 1 – Stop Drinking Alcohol

Alcohol is a dangerous poison that many of us put into our bodies on a weekly or even daily basis. The harmful effects of alcohol include:

1. **Anemia:** Alcohol damages the red blood cells that transport oxygen around your body and this can lead to anemia – a condition that causes you to have an abnormally low red blood cell count. The symptoms of anemia include difficulty breathing, pale skin and tiredness.
2. **Brain Damage:** Drinking alcohol shrinks certain areas of your brain which can cause memory loss, impaired brain function, poor judgment and more.
3. **Cancer:** Alcohol has been directly linked with multiple types of cancer including breast cancer, colon cancer, liver cancer, mouth cancer and throat

cancer. Your risk for these cancers increases in line with the amount of alcohol you consume.

4. **Dehydration:** Alcohol often causes excessive urination and this leads to dehydration. The negative effects of dehydration include excessive thirst, impaired organ function, reduced strength levels and sleep problems.

5. **Heart Disease:** Numerous studies have highlighted the links between heavy alcohol consumption and heart disease. In addition to this, alcohol can also weaken your heart and cause irregular heartbeats.

6. **Liver Damage:** Alcohol is extremely damaging to your liver cells and can cause liver failure, liver cirrhosis (scarring of the liver) and more.

7. **Nerve Damage:** Drinking alcohol on a regular basis can lead to a specific type of nerve damage called alcoholic neuropathy. The symptoms of alcoholic neuropathy include constipation, dizziness, impotence and numbness in your arms and legs.

8. **Pancreas Damage:** Alcohol adversely affects your pancreas and can lead to pancreatitis – a disorder where your pancreas becomes inflamed. Pancreatitis is a painful disorder and can cause abdominal pain, abdominal swelling and nausea.

By eliminating alcohol, you avoid all the harmful effects listed above. However, if alcohol is something that you drink regularly, the thought of giving it up for a full month may sound impossible. The good news is that there are plenty of things you can do to make the process of quitting alcohol easier. The list below outlines some of these top tips for giving up alcohol:

1. **Tell Your Friends & Family:** If you don't tell your friends and family that you're planning to quit alcohol for the next 30 days, they'll be likely to offer you alcohol or encourage you to drink it. This adds unnecessary temptation and makes it much more difficult to stay alcohol free. By making your intentions known, you'll remove this temptation and also gain help and support from those around you. In addition, verbalizing your intent increases your commitment to it.

2. **Remove Alcohol from Your Environment:** If your home contains alcohol or you socialize in bars on a regular basis, you'll be constantly exposed to alcohol and this is another strong source of temptation. Therefore, make sure your home contains no alcohol for the duration of your 30-day detox and if you often spend time where alcohol is prominent, consider skipping them for the next month.

3. **Drink Plenty of Water:** Drinking water is a great way to stay hydrated and has countless health benefits. Additionally, many people confuse a craving for alcohol with their body craving water, so by filling up on water, you may actually feel less compelled to drink alcohol.

Habit Change 2 – Cut Out Processed Foods

Processed foods are foods that contain artificial or chemical substances. Examples of processed foods include cakes, chips, cookies, fast food and soda. Like alcohol, processed foods are a toxic substance that many people consume on a daily basis. The negative symptoms of eating processed foods regularly include:

1. **Cell & Organ Damage:** The toxins in processed foods damage your cells and vital organs which can cause them to function improperly and have numerous adverse effects on your health.
2. **Chronic Disease:** Numerous studies have shown that the artificial ingredients in processed foods can increase your risk for a range of chronic diseases including cancer, diabetes and heart disease.
3. **Digestive Problems:** In addition to their high chemical content, processed foods also contain very little fiber. This can lead to a range of digestive complaints including constipation and diarrhea.
4. **Reduced Energy Levels:** Many of the toxins in processed foods have an adverse effect on your energy levels and can leave you feeling tired, lethargic and unproductive.
5. **Weight Gain:** Processed foods are packed with calories which lead to weight gain. They also contain numerous addictive substances that make you more prone to overeating and cause further weight gain.

Avoiding processed foods for the next 30 days will protect you from the toxins they contain and significantly boost your health. If you currently eat lots of processed foods and need some help giving them up, check out the tips in the section below:

1. **Get Your Sugar from Fruits & Honey:** One of the main reasons people eat so many processed foods is that they want a sugar fix. By filling up on fruits and honey, you can satisfy your sweet tooth while also providing your body with lots of essential nutrients.

2. **Replace Fried Meat with Marinated Meat:** Fried meats are one of the most popular processed foods around. However, by marinating fresh cuts of meat in a mixture of spices and extra virgin olive oil, you can enjoy the same great taste without any toxic chemicals.

3. **Replace Chips with Roast Nuts & Seeds:** Chips are another highly addictive processed food that many people consume. By roasting your favorite nuts or seeds in extra virgin olive oil and your favorite spices, you can replicate the great taste of chips and replace their harmful ingredients with a dose of healthy fats.

4. **Replace Soda with Fruit Infused Water or Herbal Tea:** Soda is one of the most damaging processed foods around. The good news is that there are plenty of sweet but healthy liquid alternatives to soda available including fruit infused water and herbal tea. Both these options contain no calories and no added chemical ingredients.

Habit Change 3 – Avoid the News

You may be surprised to see 'avoid the news' listed as something you should do as part of a detox program. After all, the news is something many of us tune into every day. It is often perceived as an essential and positive tool that keeps people informed and up to date and lets them know what is going on in the world around them. However, when you take a closer look at the news, it's easy to see how it can become a mental and physical toxin that has a detrimental effect on your happiness and wellbeing. The list below provides further details on how the news can be harmful to your body and mind:

1. **It's A Negative Influence:** While there are positive news stories out there, an overwhelming amount of what gets covered in the news is negative. War, terrorism, murder and corruption constantly make the headlines and get the majority of coverage in the mainstream media. This negative tone can have a detrimental effect on your outlook in life and cause you to become increasingly cynical towards other people, situations and circumstances around you.

2. **It Damages Your Body:** The negative stories that get covered in the news are designed to incite anger, fear and stress. For example, when you see a story in the news about a terrorist attack, your initial reaction is often strong anger or fear towards the people responsible for the attack. These reactions cause cortisol (the stress hormone) to be released

into your body. If the levels of cortisol in your body become excessive, they can damage your body and ultimately lead to chronic fatigue, heart disease, unbalanced blood glucose levels, weight gain, a weak immune system and more.

3. **It's Addictive:** News stories are structured in a way that leave you wanting more. If a crime is reported, you're encouraged to keep following the story to find out what happened to the people involved. If a war breaks out, you're encouraged to keep coming back to see how it develops. This can cause you to unknowingly develop an addiction to the news and become reliant on it as a daily source of fulfillment.

4. **It Wastes Your Time:** Many people don't realize how much time they spend consuming the news. However, if you spend 30 minutes each morning and evening consuming the news and then check it sporadically throughout the day in 5 or 10 minute intervals, you can easily spend an hour or more per day on the news. When you consider that many news stories are repeated and you consume very little new information while reading or watching the news, it's easy to see how this time could be used more productively.

5. **It Inhibits Your Creativity:** The news is filled with bias and agenda. Every story is reported in a way that influences your opinion and makes you think about it in a very specific way. This bias and influence from the news affects the way you think about other things in your daily life. It prevents you

from approaching tasks and projects in an objective way which has a detrimental effect on your creativity.

By stepping back from the news for the next 30 days, you'll not only free up time in your schedule but also quickly start to feel much calmer and more positive. The best way to avoid the news will depend on your own personal consumption habits. However, the list below contains some effective tips you can use to shield yourself from the news during the next 30 days:

1. **Assess Your Current News Consumption Habits:** By making a list of the times you consume the news each day and the mediums you use to consume it, you will get a better understanding of the best ways for you to avoid the news and then create an effective action plan. For example, if you realize that you watch the news on TV nightly between 6pm and 7pm, you can turn off the TV and schedule another activity during this time. If you notice that you always read the news on a certain website, you can actively avoid that website.

2. **Avoid News Conversations:** Even if you're not directly consuming the news, it's likely that there are people in your life who talk about it regularly. By identifying these people and then either telling them that you're avoiding the news for the next 30 days or shifting the conversation to a new topic, you'll cut out this indirect news source.

New Year Detox

3. **Block News Websites:** While setting the intention to avoid news websites is a good start, taking extra precautions and blocking these sites act as an extra line of defense during the times you get tempted. There are lots of apps, browser extensions and software programs available that can be used to block updates from news sites, so find one that works for you and get it installed.

4. **Cancel Your Newspaper Subscription:** If you have a newspaper subscription, it's important that you cancel it for the duration of your detox to avoid any potential temptation.

5. **Unsubscribe from News Emails:** Emails are another source that can potentially re-introduce the news into your life when you're trying to avoid it. So if you're subscribed to any emails that provide news updates, make sure you unsubscribe while you're participating in the detox.

6. **Remove News Apps from Your Smartphone & Tablet:** If you have any news apps on your smartphone or tablet, they'll need to be removed. Even if you turn off notifications from these apps, having the news just one click away is a temptation you don't want during your detox.

7. **Substitute TV News Consumption:** If you watch TV news at specific times each day, turn off the TV and choose another activity to do during this time instead. There are lots of things you can do during this time such as reading a book, going for a walk,

spending time with your friends or family or taking up a new hobby.

Habit Change 4 – Reduce Light Levels at Night

Night time light is an environmental toxin that many people fail to consider when trying to detox their bodies. However, being exposed to bright light during the last few hours of the day can have a detrimental effect on your sleep quality. In addition to this, even the smallest amount of light in the bedroom can disrupt your sleep.

The reason for this is that light suppresses the production of melatonin – a hormone that helps you sleep and boosts your sleep quality. The blue light emitted from electronic devices such as cell phones, computers and tablets is particularly harmful and reduces the production of melatonin in your body even more drastically than other types of light. Many people keep their cellphones and tablets in the bedroom and check them during the night which results in their bodies being constantly exposed to blue light.

The good news is that reducing your exposure to light and blue light during the last few hours of the day is relatively simple. To start cutting back on night time light and boosting your sleep quality, follow the top tips below:

1. **Dim or Turn Off the Lights:** To get your body ready for sleep and to stimulate the production of melatonin, you'll want to reduce the overall light

levels in your environment 3-4 hours before you sleep. If you don't need the lights for anything specific, you can turn them off completely and light a few candles instead. If you do need the lights on for a specific activity such as cooking or reading, keep them on but dim them so that the overall brightness in the room is reduced.

2. **Turn Off the TV:** The TV emits lots of bright light and if you watch it during the last few hours before you sleep, it can disrupt your sleep cycles, even if the other lights in the room are off. To avoid this disruption and ensure that you get a good night's sleep, turn off the TV 3-4 hours before you sleep. If there's something you really want to watch, record the program or use a streaming service to watch it earlier in the day.

3. **Reduce the Brightness of Your Computer, Smartphone & Tablet:** As mentioned above, the blue light that comes from computers, smartphones and tablets is highly disruptive to your sleep cycles. To minimize the harmful effects of blue light, reduce the brightness of your computer, smartphone and tablet screens 3-4 hours before you sleep. You can either do this manually or use a program such as f.lux which automates the process.

Habit Change 5 – Learn to Say No

Obligation and feeling like we should always say yes have become ingrained in our modern lives. Every day we have multiple people asking for favors or placing demands on our time and since we've been taught to feel guilty about saying no, we often say yes, regardless of how we truly feel. However, always saying yes can be seriously harmful to your mental wellbeing and have the following negative outcomes:

- **Stress:** When you're already busy and feel like you have to say yes to things that you don't really want to do, you'll feel increasingly overwhelmed and stressed. Not only does this stress damage your body but it also sucks the enjoyment out of everything you do and turns your life into a constant struggle to get things done.

- **Feeling Powerless:** If you feel like you can't say no, you'll feel powerless to the demands and requests of other people that will inevitably come your way. You'll feel like you have little or no control in your life which is incredibly draining and frustrating.

- **Resentment:** When you don't learn to say no to people, you often get in the habit of blaming them for taking up your time, even though you have complete freedom to give them your time or not. This can lead to strong, unjustified feelings of resentment towards other people, even when they're asking perfectly reasonable questions.

If you're used to saying yes to everything and everyone, starting to say no can seem like a huge step. However, it's a lot easier than it seems and once you get in the habit of saying no, you'll feel a huge sense of relief and freedom come over you. To get in the habit of saying no, follow the advice below:

- **Slow Down:** When people ask us to do something, we often feel compelled to give them an answer quickly and rush into saying yes out of guilt. However, if you don't have an answer in that moment, it's best to tell the person 'I'll let you know when I've checked my schedule' or 'I don't know yet'. They'll appreciate the honesty and it's better than giving them false expectations or rushing into something you don't want to do.

- **Feel for the Truth:** You can often find the true answer to a question by paying close attention to how you feel when it's asked. If you don't feel anything at the time, ask yourself the question again and monitor how you feel. If you initially feel excitement and enthusiasm about the request, the true answer is almost definitely a yes. If you feel apprehension or negativity towards the question, your honest answer is no.

- **Drop the Guilt:** If your true answer is no, you may start to feel guilty about not wanting to help the other person. However, telling the truth is the best option for you and them and there's no reason to feel guilty about that. By holding to the truth, you'll avoid all the stress, overwhelm and powerlessness that would have come with saying yes and they won't be on the receiving end of any negativity from you.

New Year Detox

- **Don't Justify:** Whether you say yes or no, it's completely your choice. Don't feel like you have to explain your answer to other people. If they push for an explanation of why you've said no, be honest and straight to the point. If you simply don't feel like it or you've got something else you'd prefer to do, tell them that. Most people will appreciate your honesty.

The Body and Mind Detox Blueprint – Week 2

The second week of **The Body and Mind Detox Blueprint** involves a further five habit changes which build upon the changes you made in the first week. Unlike week 1 which involved removing five things from your lifestyle, this second week removes just four things and adds in one new activity which enhances the detox process.

As with the first week, we recommend that you change one habit for each of the first five days and then spend the final two days reinforcing these habits. However, if you have an alternative technique that you prefer, you can use that instead.

Habit Change 1 – Stop Drinking Caffeine

Caffeine is something many of us consume multiple times each day. In fact, many of us struggle to function properly without regular doses of caffeine during the day. Constantly drinking caffeine can have a number of harmful effects which are listed below:

1. **Dehydration:** Caffeine is a mild diuretic and causes you to urinate more frequently. Drinking large amounts of caffeine can compound this effect, cause you to lose large amounts of fluid during the day and contribute to mild dehydration.

2. **Digestive Problems:** Research has shown that drinking caffeine on an empty stomach increases your risk for indigestion and stomach pain.

3. **Headaches:** Persistent caffeine consumption has been linked with daily chronic headaches. In addition to this, caffeine withdrawal can cause headaches and migraines in people who consume it daily.

4. **High Blood Pressure:** Numerous studies have shown that caffeine can raise your blood pressure. Increased blood pressure damages your blood cells and vital organs and also increases your risk of heart disease and stroke.

5. **Sleep Problems:** Caffeine is a stimulant and makes you more alert. While this alertness can be useful during the day, it can also disrupt your sleep patterns and make it difficult to fall asleep at night.

Cutting caffeine out of your lifestyle may seem like a huge change. However, there are a number of things you can do to make ditching caffeine easier and these are outlined in the list below:

1. **Try Fruit & Herbal Teas:** Fruit and herbal teas are a fantastic caffeine free alternative to coffee and caffeinated teas such as black tea and green tea. There are lots of different flavors to choose from and you're sure to find at least one fruit or herbal tea that you love.

2. **Drink More Water:** Some people find that withdrawal from caffeine causes them to become

fatigued and dehydrated. By drinking more water, you'll instantly alleviate these symptoms and also keep your hands and mouth occupied during the times you'd usually be chugging down caffeine.

3. **Pack Healthy Snacks:** Coffee and tea can help to alleviate any hunger you experience between meals, so you may find that your appetite increases after giving them up. By packing healthy snacks such as fruit, nuts and seeds, you'll be prepared for any hunger cravings if they strike.

4. **Walk Daily:** Walking is a simple but effective activity that will help to boost your alertness and take your mind off any feelings of caffeine withdrawal. Just 15 minutes each day will make a huge difference and make giving up coffee much easier.

Habit Change 2 – Cut Out Dairy

Dairy is something that more and more people are starting to cut back on. The reason for this is that too much dairy can be very harmful to the body. The section below outlines the main ways that dairy can damage your health:

1. **It Causes Inflammation in The Body:** Dairy causes huge amounts of inflammation in the body. This can lead to digestive problems, skin problems, pain, swelling and more.

2. **It Increases Acidity in The Body:** Dairy products are highly acidic and disrupt the neutral pH balance in your body. This increased acidity damages your body in various ways and can cause allergies,

weaken your bones and increase your risk for a number of chronic diseases.

3. **It's Packed Full of Hormones:** Milk contains an average of 60 different hormones including the genetically engineered growth hormone – rBGH (recombinant bovine growth hormone). These hormones have been linked with cancer and a range of other chronic diseases.

4. **It's Packed Full of Antibiotics:** The hormones that cows are injected with cause a range of health problems including udder infections and udder inflammation. These infections are then treated with antibiotics which make their way into the dairy products you consume. These antibiotics are harmful to humans and can weaken your immune system, damage your body's cells and vital organs and much more.

5. **It's Packed Full of Chemicals:** Most dairy products are highly processed and packed full of dangerous chemicals including aspartame and sucralose. These chemicals have a long list of negative side effects and have been shown to significantly increase your risk for cancer, diabetes, mood problems and seizures.

Ditching dairy may seem daunting if it's something you're used to consuming on a daily basis. However, the following guidelines can be used to help you ease into the process:

1. **Try Dairy Free Milks:** There are lots of dairy free milks out there which taste great and are packed full

of nutrition. Some of the most popular types of dairy free milk include almond milk, cashew milk, coconut milk and hazelnut milk.

2. **Try Nut Cheese:** Nut cheese contains no dairy or soy and is a fantastic healthy alternative to dairy packed cheese. There are plenty of online stores which sell a range of tasty nut cheeses and also hundreds of recipes online that you can use to make your very own nut cheeses.

3. **Replace Butter with Olive Oil:** Olive oil is a brilliant alternative to butter that can be used for cooking and spreading. Not only does it contain zero dairy but it's also packed full of healthy fats which support your body and allow it to perform optimally.

4. **Check the Ingredients Lists on Your Foods:** Butter, cheese, milk and yogurt are all obvious sources of dairy that you should avoid. However, many foods that you wouldn't expect to contain dairy actually do. Some of the top food sources of hidden dairy include breath mints, chewing gum, chicken broth and processed meats. This hidden dairy can be listed as many different ingredients including buttermilk, calcium caseinate, casein, curds, custard, cream, lactalbumin, lactoferrin, lactoglobulin, lactose, milk powder, milk solids, whey and zinc caseinate.

Habit Change 3 – Avoid Social Media

When used in moderation, social media is a great tool that allows us to stay connected with friends and family members. However, many people spend an hour or more

New Year Detox

each day connected to Facebook, Twitter and other social networks. This constant connection to social media can have the following harmful effects on your mind:

1. **Addiction:** With instant social media notifications now available on smartphones, it has become highly addictive. When a social media notification pops up, you probably feel like you have to respond to it instantly, regardless of what you're doing at the time. If you go for a few hours without checking your Facebook or Twitter account, you'll likely feel a strong craving to do so. Allowing social media to have so much control over your actions and feelings is not good and can cause you to become dependent on it.

2. **Distraction:** Social media can become highly distracting and prevent you from fully focusing on what you're doing in that moment. Many people can't eat a meal, have a face to face conversation or enjoy a movie without checking their smartphone for social media updates. This detracts from your experience of that moment and makes you miss out on all the beauty life has to offer.

3. **Negativity:** If people have a bad day or bad experience, they often post about it on social media. These posts are then met with comments from other people sharing their frustrations and adding to the negativity. In fact, you've probably posted something similar many times on social media yourself without even realizing. This constant exposure to and encouragement of negativity

shapes your mind and causes you to become increasingly pessimistic about the situations in your life.

4. **Reduced Independent Thinking:** Social media is geared around agreement and acceptance. Every post includes metrics about the likes, shares or re-tweets it has received. If a post has a large number of these social media votes, you're much more likely to like, share or re-tweet it yourself, even if it's not in line with your own personal beliefs. This form of social media peer pressure indirectly affects your ability to think critically as you unknowingly become reliant on the opinions of others when making your decisions.

5. **Reduced Productivity:** Since most people connect to social media in short burst throughout the day, they don't realize how much of their time is actually being wasted. After all, it takes less than five minutes to reply to a message, check your notifications or comment on a post. However, if you sit down and add up all the time you spend on social media in a day, you'll probably find that an hour or more of your time is being lost to these social networks. Checking social media sporadically also disrupts the flow and focus you have toward the tasks you're performing at the time which further reduces your productivity.

6. **Reduced Self Esteem:** Social media gives us an unprecedented level of access into the lives of our family members, friends and acquaintances. We can

now see what they're doing at any point in time through text, photo and even video updates. However, this deep level of access can be highly damaging to your self-esteem and cause you to feel inadequate because you weren't invited to a party or because certain friends appear to be living a much better life than you.

By disconnecting from social media, you'll avoid all the noise and negativity it brings to your life and create space for positivity, peace and calm. The list below contains some top tips you can use to stay away from social media:

1. **Tell Your Friends & Family Members:** If you're often active on social media, your friends and family members may start to wonder why you've disappeared and ask why you haven't responded to their social media messages. By telling them that you're temporarily signing off from social media, they won't have these concerns and you won't be given reminders and temptations that could potentially bring you back to social media.

2. **Block Social Media Websites:** If you're used to logging into social media websites multiple times each day, the intention to stay away often isn't enough. By blocking social media websites with an app, browser extension or software program, you can avoid these sites, even if you do get tempted to try and login.

3. **Turn Off Social Media Notifications:** Social media notifications are one of the main factors that bring

you back to these sites multiple times each day. By turning off app and email social media notifications, you won't be given any potentially tempting updates and staying away will be much easier.

4. **Remove Social Media Apps from Your Smartphone & Tablet:** Apps are another tool that can potentially bring you back to social media when you're trying to avoid it. By removing them from your smartphone and tablet, you remove the temptation to quickly click on social media sites and increase your chances of success.

Habit Change 4 – Reduce Night Time Noise

Night time noise is another environmental toxin that can potentially affect your sleep quality. Night time noise can come from various sources including noisy neighbors or roommates, traffic outside your home, people walking by at night or even the wind and rain banging and blowing against your doors and windows.

While it may seem like an impossible task to avoid night time noise, there are lots of things you can do to significantly reduce the volume inside your home and bedroom at night and ensure that you get a good night's sleep. The list below contains some top tips which will help you minimize the amount of night time noise you experience:

1. **Move Your Bed:** Placing your bed as far away from the source of night time noise as possible is a great way to reduce the impact it has on your sleep

patterns. For example, if you have noisy neighbors, placing your bed at the opposite side of the room to the wall you share with your neighbors will limit the amount of noise you hear. If you notice that lots of noise comes in through the window at night, placing your bed as far away from the window as possible will help to reduce the noise that reaches you.

2. **Try Acoustic Panels:** Acoustic panels are an innovative solution that absorb any sound within the room and allow you to make it instantly quieter. Acoustic panels come in many different colors and designs, so you can easily find some that match your home and get them installed.

3. **Use Window & Door Insulating Foam:** Having gaps in your windows and doors can substantially increase the amount of night time noise you experience. By using window and door insulating foam, you can seal these gaps, eliminate any noise that comes through them and enjoy a better night's sleep.

4. **Try Earplugs:** If you find that you're still being exposed to large amounts of night time noise after implementing the suggestions above, earplugs are a great way to block it out. They're cheap, effective, easy to use and mold to the shape of your ears to provide maximum comfort while you sleep.

Habit Change 5 – Spend Some Time in Nature

With our modern lives becoming increasingly busy and dependent on technology, we often spend very little time outside in nature. However, spending time in nature has countless health benefits which are highlighted in the list below:

1. **Enhanced Mood:** Nature is full of beautiful things such as animals, flowers, lakes and trees. By spending more time appreciating this beauty, your mood will naturally lift and you'll feel much happier in your day to day life.

2. **Increased Energy Levels:** Being outside in nature has a rejuvenating effect on your body and mind. If you're feeling tired, just a few minutes in nature will eliminate any fatigue and boost your energy levels.

3. **Increased Vitamin D Levels:** Vitamin D (also known as the sunshine vitamin) is produced when your skin gets exposed to sunlight. It strengthens your bones and teeth while also protecting against various chronic diseases. By getting outside, you can top up your vitamin D levels and enjoy all the benefits it provides.

4. **Reduced Stress Levels:** Nature is a peaceful and stress free environment. When you step outside into nature, you'll find that any stress you're currently experiencing quickly melts away and you'll feel much calmer and more relaxed.

New Year Detox

To maximize the benefits of nature, try and spend at least 30 minutes each day enjoying all the beauty the Earth has to offer. If 30 minutes each day sounds like a huge commitment, try implementing the suggestions below:

1. **Break It Up:** If you don't feel like you have time to spend a full 30 minutes in nature, break it up into smaller, more manageable segments that fit into your current schedule. For example, you could try spending 10 minutes in nature in the morning before you go to work, 10 minutes in nature during your lunch break and 10 minutes in nature in the evening.

2. **Use the Time You Have Gained from Detoxing:** At this point in the detox, you should have gained extra time each day by avoiding the news, giving up social media and learning to say no to people. You can use this additional time to enjoy nature and all the benefits it has to offer.

3. **Get Creative:** Enjoying nature doesn't have to mean sitting in the same spot every day and there are lots of different ways to experience the Earth's natural beauty. Cycling, exploring new trails, gardening, visiting botanical gardens, taking mini-vacations to areas of natural beauty and walking are just some of the many ways you can get out in nature.

The Body and Mind Detox Blueprint – Week 3

The third week of **The Body and Mind Detox Blueprint** removes three more things from your lifestyle while also adding two new positive habits. Like the previous weeks, our recommended approach is to implement one change for each of the first five days then spend the last two days perfecting these changes. However, feel free to use any technique that allows you to successfully master the five habit changes within the week.

Habit Change 1 – Cut Out Grains & Starch

Grains and starches have become a dominant part of our modern diets. For a long time people believed that grains and starches were a healthy, nutritious source of carbohydrates that should be eaten daily. However, more recent studies have highlighted the dangers of these foods and the many ways they damage our bodies. The list below outlines the negative effects of eating grains and starches:

1. **Unstable Blood Glucose Levels:** Grains causes your blood glucose levels to constantly spike and then crash. This results in your energy levels being extremely unstable and also damages your body's cells and vital organs.

2. **Toxic Ingredients:** Grains are loaded with dangerous gluten, lectins and phytic acid. Gluten can cause bloating, diarrhea and stomach pain while lectins damage your stomach lining and phytic acid

New Year Detox

prevents your body from absorbing many of the essential nutrients in your foods.

Eliminating grains from your diet allows you to avoid these toxic ingredients and their harmful effects. However, if you eat grains on a regular basis, this may sound like a huge sacrifice. Fortunately, with the right approach, giving up grains isn't as difficult as it seems. The section below contains some top tips you can use to make the transition to a grain free diet as easy as possible:

1. **Be Aware of The Side Effects:** Grains contain high levels of carbohydrates which are your body's preferred energy source. As a result, you may experience periods of low energy and concentration for the first few days after giving up on grains.

2. **Increase Your Intake of Fruits & Vegetables:** Fruits and vegetables are a healthy, nutritious source of carbohydrates that you can use to supplement the carbs you lose by ditching grains. Many fruits and vegetables can also be used to create healthy alternatives to your favorite grain based foods. For example, regular rice can be replaced with cauliflower rice and spaghetti squash strands can be used as an alternative to regular spaghetti.

3. **Experiment with Grain Free Recipes:** Grain free recipes taste incredible and once you've tried them, you probably won't even miss grains because they taste so good. There are thousands of free high quality grain free recipes online.

4. **Try Grain Free Flours:** Grain free flours such as almond flour and coconut flour are an excellent cooking ingredient that allow you to enjoy breads, cakes, cookies and more without adding grain to your diet.

Habit Change 2 – Limit Internet Activity

The Internet is something we rely on every day for communication, shopping and work. There's no denying that it's an incredibly useful and valuable tool but like the news and social media, the Internet can be a huge source of distraction, mental noise and stress if you're always connected. The section below discusses how the Internet can reduce your physical and mental wellbeing when overused:

1. **Addiction:** Internet addiction is a very real problem with many people feeling strong feelings of withdrawal whenever they are unable to connect. This addiction can have a strong negative and control your actions and feelings in ways that aren't beneficial to you.

2. **Distraction:** Being connected to the Internet can distract you in hundreds of different ways. If you receive an email, you often stop what you're doing to check and respond to it. If you're reading an article online, there are multiple adverts and links on the page designed to grab your attention. This makes it very hard to fully focus on one thing when connected to the Internet and prevents you from living in the moment.

3. **Increased Stress:** The constant connectivity provided by the Internet has created a culture where people expect fast, almost instantaneous responses to their messages and emails at any time of day or night. This expectation can be extremely stressful as you never feel you can fully relax and disconnect from the Internet. As mentioned throughout this eBook, stress is harmful to both your body and mind. It causes the stress hormone cortisol to be released into the body which can damage many of your cells and vital organs and also makes it impossible to feel calm and at peace.

4. **Reduced Critical Thinking:** While the Internet is a fantastic source of information, the ease of access to this information can be detrimental to your ability to think critically and independently. Every time you have a question or need to do some research, it's likely that you log onto the Internet and regurgitate the information you find without questioning its accuracy or authenticity. Over time you become reliant on the Internet for this information and it destroys your ability to think critically and objectively.

5. **Reduced Productivity:** The constant connection to the Internet combined with the feeling that you need to respond to any emails or messages quickly often has a negative effect on your productivity. If you're using the Internet for research or other online tasks, distractions such as adverts, emails and other websites often get the better of you which

results in the task taking much longer than it should. Even if you're performing offline tasks, being connected to the Internet via your smartphone can easily take you away from them and disrupt your focus and productivity towards the tasks at hand.

To avoid the negative consequences of heavy Internet use, you need to limit your Internet activity. This doesn't mean disconnecting from the Internet completely but it does mean cutting down your usage, so that you're only using the Internet for essential tasks. The section below provides you with some helpful advice you can use to moderate your Internet usage:

1. **Check Email in Batches:** We usually keep our emails open all day, then check and respond to them as they come in. By checking your emails at set times each day and then using this time to fully focus on reading and responding to them, you'll spend much less time on emails overall.

2. **Set an Intention to Focus Fully on Each Task:** When we don't focus fully on the task we're performing, our mind wanders and we're more likely to get distracted. If you set an intention to stay focused on the task and be vigilant, you'll get it done much faster and only use the Internet when necessary.

3. **Try the Pomodoro Technique:** The Pomodoro technique is a fantastic way to stay focused and maximize your productivity. It involves working for 25 minutes and then having a short five minute break. The regular breaks help to constantly refresh

and rejuvenate your mind while the intense focus you get from working in 25 minute intervals increases the speed with which you get things done. You can get started with the Pomodoro technique right now by checking out Tomato-Timer.com.

4. **Use a Browser Blocker:** A browser blocker will keep you away from any potentially distracting and time wasting websites while still allowing you to access the sites you need for any research or tasks.

5. **Disconnect from the Internet in the Morning and Evening:** Many of us have become accustomed to connecting to the Internet as soon as we wake up and then staying connected to the Internet right up until we sleep. By disconnecting from the Internet for the first hour of each morning and the last three or four hours of each evening, you can break this cycle and reduce your reliance on the Internet. Knowing that you're going to be disconnecting from the Internet at certain times each day will increase your productivity and force you to use the time you spend connected to the Internet efficiently. Additionally, it will improve your mental wellbeing as it will create time and space for you to relax and completely take your focus away from the constant connectivity of the Internet.

Habit Change 3 – Add Green Smoothies to Your Diet

Green smoothies are a fantastic source of nutrition, 100% free from toxins and taste delicious. They're also an excellent detox tool and help to cleanse your body in the following ways:

1. **Easy to Digest:** Green smoothies are blended and liquefied before they reach your stomach. This makes them much easier to digest than solid foods and gives your digestive system an opportunity to rest and replenish without you missing out on any valuable nutrition.

2. **High Fiber Content:** The fruits and vegetables in green smoothies add large amounts of fiber to your day. Fiber boosts your digestive health and also helps to flush harmful toxins out of your digestive tract.

3. **High Vitamin & Mineral Content:** Green smoothies are packed full of vitamins and minerals. These essential nutrients support the vital organs in your body which are responsible for eliminating toxins and ensure that they're removed from your body quickly and efficiently.

4. **High Water Content:** Water is the main ingredient in green smoothies and helps to further detoxify your body by flushing toxins out of your skin and internal organs.

To get the best results with green smoothies, replace one of your meals with a green smoothie each day. There are countless green smoothie recipes available online which you can use to start enjoying all the benefits they offer. However, we've outlined five green smoothie recipes to get you started below. Each recipe yields two servings:

New Year Detox

A 30-Day Body and Mind Detox Blueprint

1. Apple & Kale Green Smoothie

Ingredients

- 4 ice cubes
- 2 cups of kale
- 1 cup of coconut water
- 1 large green apple (cored and chopped)
- 1 small stalk of celery

Instructions

1. Add all the ingredients to a blender and then blend until smooth.
2. Once the ingredients are smooth, pour the mixture into two large glasses and enjoy.

2. Kale, Pineapple & Mint Green Smoothie

Ingredients

- 4 ice cubes
- 2 cups of kale
- 1 cup of coconut water
- 1 cup of pineapple chunks
- ¼ cup of fresh mint leaves

Instructions

1. Add all the ingredients to a blender and then blend until smooth.
2. Once the ingredients are smooth, pour the mixture into two large glasses and enjoy.

New Year Detox

3. Cucumber, Ginger & Pear Green Smoothie

Ingredients

- 4 ice cubes
- 2 cups of cucumber slices
- 1 cup of coconut water
- 1 large green pear (chopped and cored)
- 1 small piece of finely grated ginger

Instructions

1. Add all the ingredients to a blender and then blend until smooth.
2. Once the ingredients are smooth, pour the mixture into two large glasses and enjoy.

4. Spinach & Strawberry Green Smoothie

Ingredients

- 4 ice cubes
- 2 cups of spinach
- 1 cup of coconut milk
- 1 cup of strawberries

Instructions

1. Add all the ingredients to a blender and then blend until smooth.
2. Once the ingredients are smooth, pour the mixture into two large glasses and enjoy.

5. Spinach & Mango Green Smoothie

Ingredients

- 4 ice cubes

- 2 cups of spinach
- 1 cup of coconut milk
- 1 cup of mango chunks

Instructions

1. Add all the ingredients to a blender and then blend until smooth.
2. Once the ingredients are smooth, pour the mixture into two large glasses and enjoy.

For more smoothie recipes and other free offers, sign up at

https://agingslowdown.com/stay-informed-with-aging-slowdown-offers/

Habit Change 4 – Try Aromatherapy

Aromatherapy is a deeply relaxing practice that involves inhaling essential oils. Not only do these essential oils smell amazing but they also help you detox mentally and physically in the following ways:

1. **Enhanced Digestive Health:** Many essential oils boost your digestive system and help it to eliminate toxins from your body faster and more efficiently.
2. **Improved Breathing:** Certain essential oils such as eucalyptus oil cleanse your lungs and open up your airways. Not only does this help to relieve congestion but it also improves the performance of your respiratory system and allows you to enjoy deeper, fuller breathing.
3. **Improved Circulation:** Many essential oils promote circulation and help to improve the flow of blood

around your body. Since the blood is responsible for carrying toxins away from your body's cells and vital organs, this enhanced circulation helps to boost the detox process.

4. **Reduced Stress Levels:** Essential oils have a soothing, relaxing effect and can make any stress you're experiencing melt away instantly. This makes them one of the most effective tools available for detoxing your mind and also protects against any physical damage caused by stress.

To get the most out of aromatherapy, buy an essential oils starter kit and then find the scents you like. Some great essential oils to start with include eucalyptus oil, lavender oil, lemon oil, peppermint oil, rosemary oil and tea tree oil, so try and get a starter kit that includes one or more of these oils. Once you've purchased the oils, you can enjoy their scents and detoxing properties in the following ways:

1. **Essential Oils Bath:** Run yourself a hot bath and then add 10 drops of your preferred essential oils so that their scents diffuse into the room as you enjoy your bath.
2. **Essential Oils Compress:** Add five drops of your preferred essential oils to a clean, damp cloth and then apply it to your skin.
3. **Essential Oils Diffusers:** Place a diffuser in each room of your house, add the required amounts of your preferred essential oils to the diffuser and then it will slowly disperse them into the air in the rooms as you go about your day.

4. **Essential Oils Pillow:** Add five drops of your preferred essential oils to a piece of tissue just before you sleep and then place this tissue under your pillow to inhale the essential oils while enjoying a good night's rest.

5. **Essential Oils Steam Inhalation:** Fill a bowl with boiling water, then add five drops of your preferred essential oils to the bowl, cover your head with a large towel, close your eyes, hold your head above the water and inhale the steam.

Habit Change 5 – Go to Bed at a Fixed Time

Sleeping at different times each night disrupts your body's sleep cycles and affects the production of melatonin. This makes it more difficult for you to fall asleep at night and has a detrimental effect on your sleep quality. Getting into a consistent bedtime routine stabilizes your sleep cycles and melatonin production. When combined with the reduction of light levels and night time noise, this allows you to maximize your sleep quality and enjoy the following benefits:

1. **Enhanced Detox:** Sleep provides all your body's cells and vital organs with an opportunity to rest and replenish. By getting higher quality sleep more consistently, your body's cells are able to remove toxins more efficiently while you detox.

2. **Improved Immunity:** Your immune system protects against a range of harmful toxins which can cause disease, infection and illness. High quality sleep

boosts your immune system and maximizes its protective properties.

3. **Reduced Inflammation:** Numerous studies have linked poor quality sleep with higher levels of inflammatory proteins in the blood. These inflammatory proteins damage your body's cells and vital organs which increases your risk for various chronic diseases and can also cause pain, redness and swelling in specific areas of the body. A consistent sleep cycle which promotes high quality sleep protects against these toxins and all their harmful effects.

4. **Reduced Stress Levels:** The quality of your sleep has a direct impact on your stress levels. Going to bed at a fixed time and improving your sleep quality helps to lower your stress levels and keep this harmful toxin out of your life.

If you're used to sleeping at different times each night, trying to switch to a fixed sleep cycle can seem difficult. However, there are lots of things you can do to smooth this transition and by following the top tips below, you'll be able to easily adjust to a fixed bedtime in just a few days:

1. **Slow Down 30 Minutes Before You Sleep:** Many people are constantly focused on another activity such as work right up until they sleep. Then when they go to bed, their mind is still highly active and this makes it difficult for them to sleep. By slowing down and dedicating the last 30 minutes of your day to unwinding and stopping thinking, you'll find it

much easier to sleep when you get in bed. To do this, simply stop any activity that you're doing 30 minutes before you sleep, turn off all your electronic devices, eliminate any distractions, be still and enjoy the moment. If any thoughts come, don't push them away but also don't give them your attention. Just focus fully on the stillness and peace of that moment.

2. **Try Herbal Teas:** There are lots of herbal teas available that are specifically designed for sleep and relaxation. By drinking one of these during the last hour before you get into bed, you'll be able to drift into a restful sleep much more quickly.

3. **Stay in Bed:** When people struggle to sleep, they often get out of bed and do something else. By staying in bed, you'll keep your focus fully on sleep and get your mind and body in the habit of being in bed at a specific time. Even if you struggle to sleep for the first few days of the transition, the habit of staying in bed will make it much easier to stabilize your sleep cycles long term.

4. **Don't Get Distracted:** In addition to getting out of bed when they can't sleep, many people stay in bed but reach for electronic devices or start talking to their partner. However, this can be just as disruptive to your sleep cycles as getting out of bed. Therefore, make sure you stay vigilant and keep your full focus on sleep while you're in bed and avoid any other distractions.

The Body and Mind Detox Blueprint – Week 4

The fourth week of **The Body and Mind Detox Blueprint** is the most intensive week of the program and involves removing two things from your lifestyle and incorporating three new things that will enhance the detox process. As with the first three weeks, we suggest that you change one habit each day for the first five days and then use the final two days to practice and perfect these habits. However, if you have a technique that you prefer, go with that.

Habit Change 1 – Cut Out Meat

Meat contains high levels of healthy fats, proteins, vitamins and minerals and is definitely not something that you should permanently eliminate from your diet. However, eating large amounts of meat for a prolonged period of time can have the following harmful effects on your body:

1. **Production of Toxins:** Eating too much meat can cause a range of harmful toxins such as acrolein, glyoxal and malondialdehyde to be produced in your body. These toxins damage your body's cells and vital organs, increase your risk for various chronic disease and are detrimental to both your physical and mental performance.

2. **Reduced Digestive Performance:** Meat is one of the most difficult foods for your body to digest and over time, it can have a negative impact on your digestive

New Year Detox

health. Not only does this reduce the amount of nutrition your digestive system extracts from the foods you eat but it also increases the amount of toxins that accumulate in your digestive tract.

By having a temporary break from meat, you can avoid all these unpleasant effects. The list below contains some top tips you can implement to help you give up meat:

1. **Eat More Fish:** Fish is a nutrient packed food that many people don't eat enough of. It's just as versatile as meat and is packed full of protein, healthy fats and a high concentration of vitamins and minerals. It's also just as versatile as meat and can be eaten on its own, with a range of different vegetables or as part of a casserole or stew.

2. **Experiment with New Vegetables:** If you currently eat a limited amount of vegetables, the thought of giving up meat in favor of vegetables probably doesn't sound very appealing. However, giving up meat provides you with the perfect opportunity to broaden your diet and try new and exciting vegetables. There are hundreds of tasty and delicious veggies you can try, so set an intention to try at least one new vegetable each day while you're meat free and enjoy all the wonderful flavors they have to offer.

3. **Try Meat Free Recipes:** There are thousands of healthy, natural, meat free recipes online including no meat alternatives to many of your favorite meals. Give them a try, find some that you like and then

keep experimenting with new recipes so that you don't get bored.

Habit Change 2 – Stop Watching TV

Like the Internet and social media, TV can be a great source of entertainment that allows you to unwind and relax when used in moderation. However, if you watch hours of TV every day, it can transform into a mental toxin that with many harmful effects. The negative effects of watching too much TV are highlighted below:

1. **Addiction:** Like most forms of media, TV can be highly addictive and you can become reliant on watching TV every day for fulfilment.
2. **Distraction:** Many people have the TV on in the background while they work, eat and have conversations with others. This constant exposure to the TV is incredibly distracting and has a negative effect on the quality of your work, your conversations with others and your enjoyment of the foods you eat.
3. **Limited Independent Thinking:** Almost all TV shows are full of bias and opinion. When you're consuming this bias and opinion for hours each day, it starts to shape the way you think and prevents you forming your own opinions.
4. **Reduced Productivity:** As mentioned above, most people have the TV on while they work and this has a detrimental effect on your productivity. Tasks take twice as long as they should because you're splitting your focus between your work and the TV.

5. **Reduced Self Esteem:** The TV is constantly filled with images of how you should look, how you should act, how you should think and how you should live your life. Being exposed to these images on a long-term basis can cause you to feel inadequate and hurt your self-esteem if you believe you're not living up to them.

Having a week where you don't watch TV will prevent all the unpleasant effects above and create a huge amount of time in your schedule. If you need some help giving up TV, you can follow the top tips below:

1. **Record Your Favorite TV Shows:** If there are any shows you really don't want to miss while you're TV free, simply record them and then watch them after you've completed your detox. This will make the thought of giving up TV much easier as you won't be permanently missing out on any shows you love.

2. **Make Meals a Focal Point:** As mentioned previously, many people eat with the TV on which then takes their attention away from the flavor and texture of the foods they're eating. When you give up TV, you can focus fully on the foods you eat and make mealtimes more pleasurable and fulfilling. This will become like a brand-new experience that's fresh, fun and exciting. You'll quickly forget about TV as you become more engaged with focusing on your food and enjoying the experience of eating.

3. **Take Up a New Activity:** Giving up TV is going to free up a significant amount of your time and this extra

time is an excellent opportunity to take up a new activity. There are countless activities you can use as an alternative to TV and the exact activity you choose will depend on your own personal preferences. However, if you're looking for some suggestions to get started, crafts, learning a musical instrument or a foreign language, reading, walking or taking up a sport are all brilliant options.

4. **Work on Your Existing Goals:** If the thought of taking up a brand-new activity doesn't appeal, you can also use the TV free time to work on any of your existing goals. Now is the perfect time to start as giving up TV will open up a noticeable amount of time in your life which you can use to fully focus on your goals.

5. **Spend More Time with Your Family or Friends:** One of the biggest complaints people have is that they don't spend enough time with their family, friends and loved ones. By giving up TV, you'll create that time and be able to spend more quality moments with the important people in your life.

6. **Spend More Time in Nature:** If you're already enjoying the time spent in nature which was introduced in week 2 of the detox, you can use the time without TV to extend it and enjoy nature for even longer each day.

Habit Change 3 – Add Juices

Juices are a key part of many detox programs and for good reason. They provide your body with a concentrated source of nutrients and help it to detox in the following ways:

1. **No Digestion:** One of the biggest benefits of juices is that they require no digestion. This gives your digestive system a complete rest and allows it to fully rejuvenate while still taking on essential nutrients.

2. **High Vitamin & Mineral Content:** Juices contain even more vitamins and minerals than green smoothies. These nutrients enhance the health of all your cells and vital organs and help them to eliminate toxins from your body with maximum efficiency.

3. **High Water Content:** Juices also contain a higher concentration of water than smoothies. Not only does this help you stay hydrated but it also clears toxins out of your system.

To start enjoying the full benefits of juicing, simply switch one of your regular meals for juice. This will mean each day you should now be eating one whole food meal, one green smoothie as a meal and one portion of juice as a meal. As with green smoothies, there are lots of fantastic juice recipes online but we've provided you with five simple and effective juice recipes below to get started. Each recipe yields two servings:

New Year Detox

A 30-Day Body and Mind Detox Blueprint

1. Beet, Berry & Carrot Juice

Ingredients

- 2 large beets
- 2 large carrots
- 1 cup of blueberries
- 1 cup of strawberries

Instructions

1. Juice all the ingredients in a juicer.
2. When the juice is ready, pour it into two large glasses and enjoy.

2. Cranberry, Cucumber, Pear & Spinach Juice

Ingredients

- 2 cups of spinach
- 1 large cucumber
- 1 cup of cranberries
- 1 large pear

Instructions

1. Juice all the ingredients in a juicer.
2. When the juice is ready, pour it into two large glasses and enjoy.

3. Green Juice

Ingredients

- 2 medium stalks of celery
- 2 cups of kale
- 1 cup of green grapes
- 1 large green apple

New Year Detox

Instructions

1. Juice all the ingredients in a juicer.
2. When the juice is ready, pour it into two large glasses and enjoy.

4. Green Leaf, Pineapple & Watermelon Juice

Ingredients

- 2 cups of lettuce
- 2 cups of watercress
- 1 cup of pineapple chunks
- 1 cup of watermelon chunks

Instructions

1. Juice all the ingredients in a juicer.
2. When the juice is ready, pour it into two large glasses and enjoy.

5. Red Juice

Ingredients

- 2 large tomatoes
- 2 large carrots
- 1 cup of mango chunks
- 1 large orange

Instructions

1. Juice all the ingredients in a juicer.
2. When the juice is ready, pour it into two large glasses and enjoy.

Sign up to get more juice recipes and other free products at

Habit Change 4 – Try Meditation

Meditation is one of the best tools for detoxing your mind and eliminating stress and negative emotions. Just a few minutes of meditation each day will give you a fresh perspective and provide you with a lasting sense of calm, peace and bliss. The section below highlights exactly how meditation enhances your mental wellbeing:

1. **Better Perspective:** One of the biggest benefits of meditation is that it stops you basing how you feel on external circumstances. By going deep within and fully connecting with your body and mind, you'll experience a state of bliss that isn't based on anything external. This allows you to feel happy, whole and fulfilled, regardless of what is going on around you.

2. **Enhanced Creativity:** Regular meditation fully opens up your mind to inspiration. This gives you access to your most creative, exciting and innovative thoughts and ideas.

3. **Improved Concentration Levels:** Meditation teaches you to stop thinking and allows you to focus intensely without any distracting thoughts getting in the way. This skill stays with you outside of meditation and allows you to concentrate quickly and easily when necessary.

4. **Reduced Stress:** When you meditate daily, stress and negativity melts away from your daily life. Not

only does this make you feel much calmer and more relaxed but it also protects your body from the harmful effects of stress.

5. **Increased Positivity:** By eliminating stress and negativity, meditation creates a space where only positive thoughts and feelings can exist. These feelings last far beyond each meditation and make you feel much happier and more fulfilled during your everyday life.

To get the most out of meditation, start meditating for 15 minutes each day. You can complete your meditations during the time you spend in nature or carve out a separate time each day if you prefer. The section below contains some helpful tips you can use to get started with meditation:

1. **Choose a Time and Stick to It:** By creating a specific intention to meditate, you're less likely to make excuses or skip meditations. You'll also find that by meditating at a consistent time each day, it quickly becomes part of your regular routine.

2. **Eliminate All Distractions:** External distractions make meditating very difficult. Therefore, you want to meditate somewhere where you're alone and there is very little noise. You should also turn off any potentially distracting electronic devices such as your smartphone.

3. **Find a Position that You're Comfortable with:** Most photos of meditation show people sitting in the lotus position (eyes closed, legs crossed, hands

resting on your knees, thumb and index finger touching in a circular shape). However, meditation can be performed in any position, so if you find the lotus position uncomfortable, try sitting on a chair, lying down or anything else that you find comfortable.

4. **Focus on Your Breaths:** Once you're in a position that you're comfortable with, begin the meditation by focusing fully on your breathing. Fully feel how each breath enters and leaves your body and how your body moves and responds to the breaths.

5. **Don't Judge Your Thoughts:** If your mind starts to wander and thoughts start to come during the meditation, be aware of them but don't judge them. Try to refocus on your breathing but don't push the thoughts away. Just observe them and let them be without any positive or negative judgment. Do this for 15 minutes and then complete the meditation.

6. **Don't Judge the Meditation:** Sometimes meditation is a smooth experience with very little thought where you are able to fully connect with your inner self and find deep peace. Other times, the thoughts come constantly and you find yourself unable to stop judging them. Both of these are fine and every meditation is unique. As long as you maintain a judgment free zone, your meditations will become increasingly beneficial and fulfilling.

Habit Change 5 – Start A Daily Gratitude List

Practicing gratitude is incredibly beneficial but something many of us neglect. There are so many good things in our life that we can appreciate but we often get caught up focusing on the negatives and the things we want to change. By practicing gratitude daily, you can cleanse your mind and enjoy the following benefits:

1. **Better Perspective:** By practicing gratitude, you'll naturally see the positives in every situation. This is an extremely valuable skill as it gives you the power to feel happy, regardless of what's going on around you.

2. **Enhanced Relationships:** Gratitude can remove the toxicity from all your relationships and allow them to blossom. By removing any negativity and showing people the appreciation they deserve, your relationships will reach a new level and be incredibly fulfilling.

3. **Increased Happiness:** Appreciation is one of the most powerful and fulfilling emotions you can experience. By actively practicing gratitude, you'll feel this positive emotion more often and this will boost your overall happiness levels.

4. **Reduced Negativity:** By increasing the amount of happiness in your life, you also reduce the amount of negativity. This means that emotions such as anger, frustration, jealousy and resentment will

slowly disappear and you'll be left with only joyful emotions.

5. **Reduced Stress:** As your happiness increases and your negativity decreases, you'll find that stress becomes a thing of the past. Your life will become constantly relaxing and blissful which has a positive effect on both your body and mind.

There are lots of ways you can incorporate gratitude into your life but one of the easiest and most effective is to start a daily gratitude list. To start a daily gratitude list, simply follow the advice below:

1. **Write Your Gratitude List in the Morning:** Your first thoughts shape your day. By setting aside some time every morning to write your gratitude list, you'll ensure that you start the day with positive emotions which you can then carry with you as the day progresses.

2. **Choose Five Things That You Are Grateful For:** This can be people, circumstances, opportunities, your work, your pets, nature or anything else that you love. Simply choose your top five and then write them down.

3. **Write Why You're Grateful for These Things:** Going deep into each of the five things you've chosen and writing down exactly why you love them will make you appreciate them even more and enhance your overall feelings of gratitude.

4. **Review Your List After Writing It:** Once you've written down the five things you're grateful for that

New Year Detox

day and why, read your list back to yourself while fully focusing on it. Feel every sentence and let the gratitude within you grow even more.

5. **Read the Gratitude List Again Before You Sleep:** Reading the gratitude list again just before you sleep will allow you to refocus on appreciation and positivity as you end the day. This provides you with a perfect platform before you sleep and helps to ensure that the gratitude will stay with you and grow as you wake up and move into the next day.

The Body and Mind Detox Blueprint – Final Two Days

The final two days of **The Body and Mind Detox Blueprint** take all the habits from the first four weeks of this program and use them to intensely cleanse your body and mind. Unlike the other parts of this detox plan where you are able to gradually implement the various habit changes, the changes for these last two days need to be implemented immediately and maintained for the entire 48 hours.

Habit Change 1 – Liquid Cleanse

The liquid cleanse is simple but challenging and involves completely avoiding all solid foods for two days and replacing your three main meals with juices. In addition to the juices, you can also keep yourself hydrated with the following drinks:

- Fruit infused water
- Fruit and herbal teas

- Water

The key benefits of this liquid cleanse phase are listed below:

1. **No Toxins:** The biggest benefit of the liquid cleanse is that since you're not eating any solid foods, you won't ingest any toxins. This has a huge rejuvenating effect on all your body's cells and vital organs.

2. **No Digestion:** By consuming just juices and fluids for two days, your digestive system will get a complete 48-hour break. This has a significant restorative effect and will notably improve the efficiency, performance and health of your digestive tract in the long term.

3. **High Vitamin & Mineral Content:** The combination of drinking large amounts of vitamins and minerals through juice while not consuming any harmful toxins accelerates the detox process and thoroughly cleanses your body during these two days.

4. **High Water Content:** When you drink just juices and liquids while avoiding solid foods for an entire two days, your body becomes incredibly hydrated and this completely flushes any remaining toxins out of your system.

5. **Weight Loss:** Juices contain very few calories while fruit infused water, fruit and herbal teas and water all contain zero calories. As a result, you'll be able to lose a notable amount of weight and lower your body fat percentage during this 48-hour liquid cleanse.

New Year Detox

Habit Change 2 – Mind Cleanse

The mind cleanse involves completely disconnecting from technology and other people for two days and using this time to relax and empty your mind. The section below contains a full list of what's required to successfully complete this 48 hour mind cleanse:

1. **No Electronics:** In order to fully empty your mind, it's important that you completely avoid all forms of electronic technology. This means no computers, smartphones, tablets, news, Internet, social media, TV or other types of electronics can be used during these two days. If electronics are a necessary for your work, you can either make sure you complete the mind cleanse during the weekend or use some vacation days to get it done without interfering with your work.

2. **No People:** This may sound extreme but other people are often one of the major causes of stress in our lives. By taking two days to be completely alone, you can reach a level of mental calmness and clarity which is almost impossible to achieve when other people are constantly present. If you live alone, you can let people that you're in touch with regularly know what you're doing so that they won't contact you or expect you to contact them. If you live with others, take a mini-vacation to somewhere that allows you to be alone for 48 hours.

3. **Spend At Least One Hour Per Day In Nature:** When you disconnect from electronics and other people

during the final two days of this detox, you'll have a lot of free time open up for you. By spending an hour or more of this time in nature each day, you can enjoy all its healing properties at an even deeper level and feel mentally and physically refreshed.

4. **Spend At Least One Hour Per Day Meditating:** Meditation is another fantastic activity that will help to cleanse your mind more fully during the final 48 hours of the detox. By meditating for at least one hour each day, you'll reach a state where you're completely calm, at peace and free from negativity.

5. **Spend At Least One Hour Per Day on Aromatherapy:** Aromatherapy is another amazing detox tool that you can use during your extra free time on the final two days of the detox. By increasing the amount of time you spend applying and inhaling essential oils, you'll remove plenty of toxins from your body and mind.

The mind cleanse has a huge number of benefits and these are highlighted below:

1. **No Distractions:** By being alone and disconnected from electronic technology for two days, you completely eliminate mental distractions from your environment. This leaves you free to fully focus on relaxing in the present moment without anything else entering your mental space.

2. **No Stress:** Another big benefit of this 48 hour mind cleanse is that you won't be exposed to any outside negative influences. This freedom from negativity

and stress gives you the space you need to completely clear your mind and develop a more open, positive mindset.

3. **Better Perspective:** Taking an extended break from external influences and detoxing your mind allows you to go deep within yourself and develop a better perspective on your life as a whole. These two days will transform the way you look at outside factors and prevent you from being conditional on them for happiness. You'll learn to truly love yourself and love life, regardless of what's going on around you.

4. **Enhanced Concentration Levels:** When you have no distractions around you, you'll find that it's much easier to focus your thoughts and direct them towards one thing at a time. After the two days have passed, your concentration levels will improve significantly and you'll be able to focus much more intensely in any situation.

5. **Increased Creativity:** Eliminating toxins from your mind creates the necessary space for creativity. Once your mind is fully open, you'll find that it naturally fills up with inspirational thoughts and ideas that can enhance every area of your life.

6. **Increased Happiness:** Removing stressful thoughts from your mind results in positive, joyful thoughts coming to you much more naturally. This has a huge effect on your overall happiness levels and helps you to enjoy every life experience much more deeply.

7. **Improved Energy Levels:** Negative thoughts and influences are extremely draining and can make you

feel tired and fatigued. Freeing yourself from them has a rejuvenating effect on your body and rapidly improves your energy levels.

8. **Stronger Relationships:** By spending a couple of days away from other people, you'll actually strengthen your relationships with them. When you remove negative thoughts from your mind and spend time reflecting on the people in your life, you'll discover what you truly love and appreciate about them. This will shine through in your future interactions with these people and take your relationships with them to new levels.

9. **Vitamin D:** One of the main reasons we don't get enough vitamin D in our modern lives is that we're glued to our computer or television screens. By turning them off for a couple of days and increasing the amount of time you spend in nature, you can fill up on this sunshine vitamin and enjoy all its benefits.

Printable Body and Mind Detox Blueprint Summary Charts

To make completing **The Body and Mind Detox Blueprint** easier we've put together a selection of printable summary charts that you can use to remind yourself of exactly what you need to do on each day of this program. Simply print the summary charts off, keep them with you and check them daily to stay on track as you detox.

New Year Detox

A 30-Day Body and Mind Detox Blueprint

Week 1 Summary Chart

Day	Habit Change	Tips
1	Stop Drinking Alcohol	Tell Your Friends & Family You're Not Drinking Alcohol
		Remove Alcohol from Your Environment
		Drink Plenty of Water
2	Cut Out Processed Foods	Get Your Sugar from Fruits & Honey
		Replace Fried Meat with Marinated Meat
		Replace Chips with Roast Nuts & Seeds
		Replace Soda with Fruit Infused Water Or Herbal Tea
3	Avoid the News	Assess Your Current News Consumption Habits
		Avoid News Conversations
		Block News Websites
		Cancel Your Newspaper Subscription
		Unsubscribe from News Emails
		Remove News Apps from Your Smartphone & Tablet
		Substitute TV News Consumption
4	Reduce Light Levels at Night	Dim Or Turn Off The Lights
		Turn Off The TV
		Reduce the Brightness Of Your Computer, Smartphone & Tablet

New Year Detox

A 30-Day Body and Mind Detox Blueprint

5	Learn to Say No	Slow Down
		Feel for The Truth
		Don't Justify
6	Practice the Last Five Habit Changes	
7	Practice the Last Five Habit Changes	

New Year Detox

A 30-Day Body and Mind Detox Blueprint

Week 2 Summary Chart

Day	Habit Change	Tips
1	Stop Drinking Caffeine	Try Fruit & Herbal Teas
		Drink More Water
		Pack Healthy Snacks
		Walk Daily
2	Cut Out Dairy	Try Dairy Free Milks
		Try Nut Cheese
		Replace Butter with Olive Oil
		Check the Ingredients List On Your Food
3	Avoid Social Media	Tell Your Friends & Family Members
		Block Social Media Websites
		Turn Off Social Media Notifications
		Remove Social Media Apps from Your Smartphone & Tablet
4	Reduce Night Time Noise	Move Your Bed
		Try Acoustic Panels
		Use Window & Door Insulating Foam
		Try Earplugs
5	Spend Some Time In Nature	Break It Up
		Use the Time You Have Gained from Detoxing
		Get Creative
6	Practice the Last Five Habit Changes	

New Year Detox

7	Practice the Last Five Habit Changes	

New Year Detox

A 30-Day Body and Mind Detox Blueprint

Week 3 Summary Chart

Day	Habit Change	Tips
1	Cut Out Grains & Starch	Be Aware of The Side Effects
		Increase Your Intake of Fruits & Vegetables
		Experiment with Grain Free Recipes
		Try Grain Free Flours
2	Limit Internet Activity	Check Email in Batches
		Set an Intention to Fully Focus on Each Task
		Try the Pomodoro Technique
		Use A Browser Blocker
		Disconnect from The Internet In The Morning & Evening
3	Add Green Smoothies	Get Started with the Five Green Smoothie Recipes on page 47
		Find Green Smoothie Recipes Online
4	Try Aromatherapy	Use an Essential Oils Bath
		Use an Essential Oils Compress
		Use an Essential Oils Diffuser
		Use an Essential Oils Pillow
		Use Essential Oils Steam Inhalation
5	Go to Bed At A Fixed Time	Slow Down 30 Minutes Before You Sleep
		Try Herbal Teas
		Stay in Bed
		Don't Get Distracted

New Year Detox

A 30-Day Body and Mind Detox Blueprint

6	Practice the Last Five Habit Changes	
7	Practice the Last Five Habit Changes	

New Year Detox

A 30-Day Body and Mind Detox Blueprint

Week 4 Summary Chart

Day	Habit Change	Tips
1	Cut Out Meat	Eat More Fish
		Experiment with New Vegetables
		Try Meat Free Recipes
2	Stop Watching TV	Record Your Favorite TV Shows
		Make Meals A Focal Point
		Take Up A New Activity
		Work on Your Existing Goals
		Spend More Time with Your Family or Friends
		Spend More Time in Nature
3	Add Juices	Get Started with The Five Juice Recipes on Page 61
		Find Juice Recipes Online
4	Try Meditation	Choose A Time & Stick to It
		Eliminate All Distractions
		Find A Position That You're Comfortable With
		Focus on Your Breaths
		Don't Judge Your Thoughts
		Don't Judge the Meditation
5	Start A Daily Gratitude List	Write Your Gratitude List in The Morning
		Choose Five Things That You Are Grateful For
		Write Why You're Grateful for These Things
		Review Your List After Writing It

New Year Detox

		Read the Gratitude List Again Before You Sleep
6	Practice the Last Five Habit Changes	
7	Practice the Last Five Habit Changes	

New Year Detox

Final Two Days Summary Chart

Day	Habit Change	Tips
29 & 30	Liquid Cleanse	Avoid All Solid Foods
		Drink Three Juices Per Day
		Rehydrate Regularly with Fruit Infused Water, Fruit & Herbal Teas & Water
	Mind Cleanse	No Electronics
		No People
		Spend At Least One Hour Per Day in Nature
		Spend At Least One Hour Per Day Meditating
		Spend At Least One Hour Per Day on Aromatherapy

New Year Detox

The Rest of the Books

The Series

New Year Detox is Book 1 in the Fitness Blueprint series:

1. New Year Detox
2. Clean Eating for Weight Loss
3. Beginner's Keto
4. 4 Minute Keto
5. Keto Diet + Intermittent Fasting
6. The Home Workout Bible

Each book can be read stand-alone, but as a series they lead you through a journey, starting with a detox, then learning clean eating and proceeding to the keto diet and exercise to burn fat and become the best you can be.

See the full series at Fitness Blueprint on Amazon.

Other Books

To see all of this author's books, both published and forthcoming titles and to get some free gifts, please sign up at:

https://agingslowdown.com/stay-informed-with-aging-slowdown-offers/

New Year Detox

About the Author

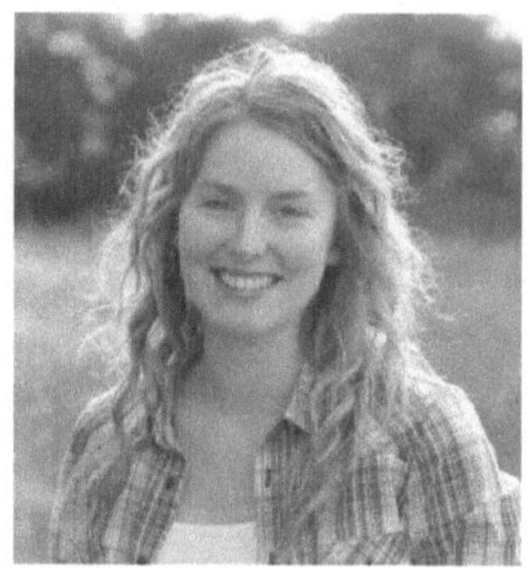

Emma Morgan is a 40 something single mother of two teenage kids.

She wakes up every morning looking forward to the day ahead. She feels relaxed, stress free and healthy. Her friends tell her she has an inner glow.

But it wasn't always like that.

After a bitter divorce that left her drained, almost broke and with two kids to support, she had too much and too little.

Too much junk food, too much stress, too much yelling, too much over-reaction. And way too much over-weight.

Too little exercise, too little sleep, too little nutrition, too little love and tolerance.

She decided to change. She decided to take control.

The result has been a journey. A personal journey into detox, exercise, weight loss, skincare and healthy living. Keto was an important part of that journey.

Along with Phil Lancaster, her 80-year-old business partner, she is the author of the anti-aging website agingslowdown.com and is passionate about helping others, both men and women, to be their happiest and healthiest selves as they approach their golden years.

New Year Detox

But this is where it all starts.

With the 30-Day Body and Mind Detox.